ALKALINE DIET:

THE BENEFITS OF EATING ALKALINE FOODS, A GUIDE FOR BEGINNERS TO HELP YOU LOSE WEIGHT, KEEP IN FORM AND LIVE A HEALTHY LIFE.

I0415160

GILLIAN WILLET

duplicate, or transmit any part of this document in either electronic means or in printed format. Recording of this publication is strictly prohibited and any storage of this document is not allowed unless with written permission from the publisher. All rights reserved.

The information provided herein is stated to be truthful and consistent, in that any liability, in terms of inattention or otherwise, by any usage or abuse of any policies, processes, or directions contained within is the solitary and utter responsibility of the recipient reader. Under no circumstances will any legal responsibility or blame be held against the publisher for any reparation, damages, or monetary loss due to the information herein, either directly or indirectly.

CONTENTS

INTRODUCTION

A lot of people have been struggling to find the best diet program fit for them. One of the most common misrepresentations these people have is their desire to lose weight. However, they fail to put vital emphasis on how to be healthy. If you want to know the best diet that is perfect for you, then you better make sure it's a healthy one, and is not destroying your body.

CHAPTER ONE

WHAT IS THE ALKALINE DIET?

The Alkaline Diet, also known as the Alkaline Acid Diet, is a diet based on the consumption of food such as fruits, vegetables, roots, nuts, and legumes, but avoiding dairy, meat, grains and salts. Recently, this diet has gained popularity among diet and nutrition specialists and authors. There is still a debate on the efficiency of alkaline diet because there is no concrete evidence that it can reduce certain diseases.

As aforementioned, fruits, vegetables, roots, nuts, and legumes are part of the alkaline diet. This is because these food release alkaline after being digested, absorbed, and metabolised. On the other hand; dairy, meat, grains and salts produce acid after they are processed. Food is categorized as acid-producing or alkaline-producing based on its pH (power of Hydrogen) values, where pH 0 - 6 is acidic, pH 8 - 14 is alkaline and pH 7 is neutral (water). Hence, the alkaline diet refers to a diet having more alkaline-producing foods.

Alkaline Diet

Our blood has a pH between 7.35 and 7.45, which is slightly alkaline. The Alkaline diet is based on the pH level of our blood and any diet that is high in acid-producing food will destroy the balance. When the body tries to revitalize the equilibrium of pH in the blood, the acidity of the food will contribute to the loss of vital minerals such as potassium, magnesium, calcium, and sodium. The imbalance will make people susceptible to illness.

Unfortunately, Western diets are more acid-producing and on it people consume few fresh fruits and vegetables. Due to the advent of the alkaline diet, the standard of the Western diet has changed considerably.

Some diet and nutrition practitioners believe that an acid-producing diet may cause some chronic illness and the following symptoms, such as:

- Headache

- Lethargy

- Frequent flu and cold, and excess mucous production

- Anxiety, nervousness

- Polycystic ovaries, ovarian cysts, benign breast cysts

Although some believe the above conditions are the result of an acid-producing diet, and the consumption of fruits and vegetables is beneficial to health, some doctors think that an acid-producing diet does not cause chronic disease. Other than that, there are proofs showing that an alkaline diets helps to prevent the formation of calcium kidney stones, osteoporosis, and age-related muscle wasting.

Surely, you have encountered an alkaline meal program somewhere online or in some reading materials. What is an alkaline diet and is this diet healthy for you? This diet all started when experts tried considering the pH level of the body.

In a person's body, the environment can be acidic or alkaline. Once the pH level is high, then the environment is alkaline. In contrary, low pH means the environment is acidic. The body does not have one single pH level, rather it can differ depending on the location. For instance, the pH level in the stomach is different from the urinary bladder.

This diet is basically all about eating foods which can promote an alkaline environment in the body while not eating foods that promote acidity to the body. What could be the reason behind this program? To start off, foods that can promote an alkaline environment in the body are considered healthy. Examples of these foods include vegetables, fruits, soy products, nuts, legumes, and cereals. If you have noticed, these foods are also rich in protein, vitamins, and minerals.

Th other principle of an alkaline diet is to avoid acidic foods because these are foods that can make your body at risk for weight gain, heart problems, kidney and liver diseases. A few of the many acidic foods include caffeine, foods with high preservatives like canned goods, sodas, fish, meat, alcohol and foods with a high sugar content. When you come to think of it, an alkaline diet is not unusual for everyone, especially when talking about a healthy diet.

Real Deal with the Alkaline Diet

According to experts, acidic foods can decrease the pH of a person's urine. When the pH is abnormally low kidney stones tend to form. To counteract this situation a person needs to increase the pH through eating alkaline rich foods, it's that simple.

Since an alkaline diet means avoiding alcohol and any other foods with high acidity, it also means you will decrease the risk of developing diseases associated with an unhealthy diet like diabetes, hypertension, and obesity. Although no exact evidences can prove this, some researchers have stated that an alkaline diet can reduce the risk of cancer.

Things to Remember

In order for the alkaline diet to work, you must condition yourself to adhere to this diet program. When it requires you to avoid unhealthy foods and drinks, then you had better do it. Water is an excellent alternative drink for soda and alcohol.

In addition, so you will not have a difficult time figuring out which are alkaline and which are acidic foods, it is best that you make a list of each category. Perhaps you can research online on what foods are rich in alkaline and those having a high acid content. Alkaline foods are not that hard to point out because the majority of foods belong to the vegetables and fruits classifications.

When you choose to eat an alkaline diet, you are actually eating foods that are very similar to what mankind was designed to eat. If you look at what our ancestors ate, you will find a diet rich in fresh fruits, vegetables, legumes, nuts, and fish. Unfortunately, man's diet today is frequently full of foods that are high in unhealthy fats, salt, cholesterol, and acidifying foods

Although some people think that man's diet changed only recently, the shift from a largely alkaline diet to an acidic diet actually began thousands of years ago. Our original diet consisted of foraged fruits, nuts and vegetables, along with whatever meat could be caught.

As soon as man started to grow his own

food, things started to change. Grains became a popular diet choice, especially after the development of stone tools. Once animals were domesticated, there were dairy products added to the diet, along with an additional amount of meat. Salt began to be added, along with sugar. The end result was a diet that was still much healthier than what many people eat today, but the shift from alkaline to acidic had begun.

It's no secret that our modern diet consists of many foods which are not healthy for us. Too much junk food and "fast food" has decreased the quality of our diet. Obesity has become the norm, and along with it a higher incidence of diseases such as diabetes, coronary disease, and cancer. If you want to improve your health and reduce the risk of many diseases, an alkaline diet can help get your body back to basics.

When foods are eaten and digested, they produce either an acidifying or alkalizing effect within the body. Some people get confused because the actual pH of the food itself doesn't have anything to do with the effect of the food once it is digested.

When more alkaline foods are consumed, the body can become slightly alkaline instead of acidic. Ideally, the blood pH level should be between 7.35 and 7.45. Foods such as citrus fruits, soy products, raw fruits and vegetables, wild rice, almonds, and natural sweeteners such as Stevia are all good alkaline food choices.

There are many benefits to shifting your

eating patterns from acidic to alkaline. When the body is kept slightly alkaline, it is less susceptible to disease. It's easier to lose weight or maintain a healthy weight level on an alkaline diet. Most people experience an increase in their energy level, as well as a lessening of anxiety and irritability once they begin eating more alkaline foods.

Mucous production is decreased and nasal congestion is reduced, making it easier to breath. Allergies are frequently alleviated as a result of an alkaline diet. The body is also less susceptible to illnesses such as cancer and diabetes. Most people find that they just feel better, with an increased sense of health and well-being, once they make a conscious effort to adhere to an alkaline diet.

The Alkaline Diet Myth

The alkaline diet is also known as the acid-alkaline diet or the alkaline ash diet. It is based around the idea that the foods you eat leave behind an "ash" residue after they have been metabolized. This ash can be acid or alkaline.

Proponents of this diet claim that certain foods can affect the acidity and alkalinity of bodily fluids, including urine and blood. If you eat foods with an acidic ash, they make the body acidic. If you eat foods with an alkaline ash, they make the body alkaline.

Acidic ash is thought to make you vulnerable to diseases such as cancer, osteoporosis, and muscle wasting, whereas alkaline ash is considered to be protective. To make sure you stay alkaline, it is recommended that you keep track of your urine using handy pH test strips.

For those who do not fully understand human physiology and are not nutrition experts, diet claims like this sound rather convincing. However, is it really true? The following will debunk this myth and clear up some confusion regarding the alkaline diet.

But first, it is necessary to understand the meaning of the pH value.

Put simply, the pH value is a measure of how acidic or alkaline something is. The pH value ranges from 0 to 14.

- 0-7 is acidic
- 7 is neutral

- 7-14 is alkaline

For example, the stomach is loaded with highly acidic hydrochloric acid, a pH value between 2 and 3.5. The acidity helps kill germs and break down food.

On the other hand, the human blood is always slightly alkaline, with a pH of between 7.35 to 7.45. Normally, the body has several effective mechanisms (discussed later) to keep the blood's pH within this range. Falling out of it is very serious and can be fatal.

Effects Of Foods On Urine And Blood pH

Foods leave behind an acid or alkaline ash. Acid ash contains phosphate and sulfur. Alkaline ash contains calcium, magnesium, and potassium.

Certain food groups are considered acidic, neutral, or alkaline. They include:

- Acidic: Meats, fish, dairy, eggs, grains, and alcohol.

- Neutral: Fats, starches, and sugars.

- Alkaline: Fruits, vegetables, nuts, and legumes.

Urine pH

Foods you eat change the pH of your urine. If you have a green smoothie for breakfast, your urine, in a few hours, will be more alkaline than if you had bacon and eggs.

For someone on an alkaline diet, urine pH can be very easily monitored and may even provide instant gratification. Unfortunately, urine pH is neither a good indicator of the overall pH of the body, nor is it a good indicator of general health.

Blood pH

Foods you eat do not change your blood pH. When you eat something with an acid ash like protein, the acids produced are quickly neutralized by bicarbonate ions in the blood. This reaction produces carbon dioxide, which is exhaled through the lungs, and salts, which are excreted by the kidneys in your urine.

During the process of excretion, the kidneys produce new bicarbonate ions, which are returned to the blood to replace the bicarbonate that was initially used to neutralize the acid. This creates a sustainable cycle in which the body is able to maintain the pH of the blood within a tight range.

Therefore, as long as your kidneys are functioning normally, your blood pH will not be influenced by the foods you eat, whether they are acidic or alkaline. The claim that eating alkaline foods will make your body or blood pH more alkaline is not true.

Acidic Diet And Cancer

Those who advocate an alkaline diet claim that it can cure cancer because cancer can only grow in an acidic environment. By eating an alkaline diet, cancer cells cannot grow, so they die.

This hypothesis is very flawed. Cancer is perfectly capable of growing in an alkaline environment. In fact, cancer grows in normal body tissue which has a slightly alkaline pH of 7.4. Many experiments have confirmed this by successfully growing cancer cells in an alkaline environment.

However, cancer cells do grow faster with acidity. Once a tumor starts to develop, it creates its own acidic environment by breaking down glucose and reducing circulation. Therefore, it is not the acidic environment that causes cancer but the cancer that causes the acidic environment.

Even more interesting is a 2005 study by the National Cancer Institute which used vitamin C (ascorbic acid) to treat cancer. They found that by administering pharmacologic doses intravenously, ascorbic acid successfully killed cancer cells without harming normal cells. This is another example of cancer cells being vulnerable to acidity, as opposed to alkalinity.

In short, there is no scientific link between eating an acidic diet and cancer. Cancer cells can grow in both acidic and alkaline environments.

Acidic Diet And Osteoporosis

Osteoporosis is a progressive bone disease characterized by a decrease in bone mineral content, leading to lowered bone density and strength and higher risk of a broken bone.

Proponents of the alkaline diet believe that in order to maintain a constant blood pH, the body takes alkaline minerals like calcium from the bones to neutralize the acids from an acidic diet. As discussed above, this is absolutely not true. The kidneys and the respiratory system are responsible for regulating blood pH, not the bones.

In fact, many studies have shown that increasing animal protein intake is positive for bone metabolism as it increases calcium retention and activates IGF-1 (insulin-like growth factor-1) that stimulates bone regeneration. Thus, the hypothesis that an acidic diet causes bone loss is not supported by science.

Acidic Diet And Muscle Wasting

Advocates of the alkaline diet believe that in order to eliminate excess acid caused by an acidic diet, the kidneys will steal amino acids (building blocks of protein) from muscle tissues, leading to muscle loss. The proposed mechanism is similar to the one causing osteoporosis.

As discussed, blood pH is regulated by the kidneys and the lungs, not the muscles. Hence, acidic foods like meats, dairy, and eggs do not cause muscle loss. As a matter of fact, they are complete dietary proteins that will support muscle repair and help prevent muscle wasting.

What Did Our Ancestors Eat?

A number of studies have examined whether our pre-agricultural ancestors ate net acidic or net alkaline diets. Very interestingly, they found that about half of the hunter-gatherers ate net acid-forming diets, while the other half ate net alkaline-forming diets.

Acid-forming diets were more common as people moved further north of the equator. The less hospitable the environment, the more animal proteins they ate. In more tropical environments where fruits and vegetables were abundant, their diet became more alkaline.

From an evolutionary perspective, the

theory that acidic or protein-rich diets cause diseases like cancer, osteoporosis, and muscle loss is not valid. Half of the hunter-gatherers were eating net acid-forming diets, yet, they had no evidence of such degenerative diseases.

It is worth noting that there is no one-size-fits-all diet that works for everyone, which is why Metabolic Typing is so helpful in determining your optimal diet. Due to our genetic variances, some people will benefit from an acidic diet, some an alkaline diet, and some some sort of diet that's in between. Thus the saying: one man's food can be another man's poison.

It is true that many people who have switched to an alkaline diet see significant health improvements.

However, do bear in mind that other reasons may be at work:

Most of us do not eat enough vegetables and fruits. According to the Center for Disease and Prevention, only 9% of Americans eat enough vegetables and 13% enough fruits. If you switch to an alkaline diet, you are automatically eating more vegetables and fruits. After all, they are very rich in phytochemicals, antioxidants, and fiber which are essential to good health. When you eat more vegetables and fruits, you are probably eating less processed foods too.

Eating less dairy and eggs will benefit those who are lactose-intolerant or have a food sensitivity to eggs, which is rather common among the general population.

Eating less grains will benefit those who

are gluten-sensitive or have leaky gut or an autoimmune disease.

Alkaline Water

One last point worth mentioning is that many people believe that drinking alkaline water (pH of 9.5 vs. pure water's pH of 7.0.) is healthier based on similar reasoning as the alkaline diet. Anyhow, it is not true. Water that is too alkaline can be detrimental to your health and lead to nutritional disequilibrium.

If you drink alkaline water all the time, it will neutralize your stomach acid and raise the alkalinity of your stomach. Over time, it will impair your ability to digest food and absorb nutrients and minerals. With less acidity in the stomach, it will also open the door for bacteria and parasites to get into your small intestine.

The bottom line is that alkaline water is not the answer to good health. Do not be fooled by marketing gimmicks. Instead, invest in a good water filtration system for your home. Clean, filtered water is still the best water for your body.

GUIDELINES

The alkaline diet is also known as the ph miracle, ph balance diet, or the acid alkaline diet, among other things. It based on the theory that everything that you eat can either cause your body to build up acid or to become more alkaline. For someone starting this diet, it can be overwhelming trying to figure out what is good (alkaline) and what is bad(acidic). This is why the alkaline diet guidelines will clear up some of the confusion.

There are many alkaline diet guidelines. The basic idea is certain substances are worse for the body then others. One of the alkaline diet guidelines is that you should attempt to eat 75-80% alkaline. Meaning that 75-80% of your diet is from the alkaline food chart.

Certain foods are considered more acid forming than others though. To give you an idea, here is a list of foods that are considered highly acid forming according to the alkaline diet guidelines: sweeteners (equal, sweet and low, nutra-sweet, and aspartame to name a few) beer, table salt, jam, ice cream, beef, lobster, fried food, processed cheese, and soft drinks. Here is a fun fact: cola has ph of 2.5. This is highly acidic. In order to neutralize one can of cola you would have to drink 32 glasses of water.

On the other side of the spectrum, there are certain food that are considered to be highly alkaline and when ingested help increase the alkalinity of the body. According to the alkaline diet guidelines, these food are as follows: sea salt, lotus rood, watermelon, tangerines, sweet potato, lime, pineapple, seaweed, pumpkin seeds, and lentils.

The alkaline diet guidelines say that drugs are extremely acid forming as well. Think about all those people who take some form of drug to ease their acid reflux. Little do they know their temporary solution is causing bigger problems for them in the long run.

There are many other alkaline diet foods

and this was just an example. The more you eat them, the better you will feel. Many times people experience a period of detoxification when they switch to the alkaline diet. The alkaline diet guidelines suggest that you go through a period of a couple of weeks in detox to rid your body of toxins and allow it to adjust to this completely new way of eating.

LIFESTYLE

The low carbohydrate and high protein diets doing the rounds these days are an invitation to bad health. All athletes know that if a fit body is to be maintained one should steer completely clear of such diets. Not only do they result in extreme fatigue, they are also are a disaster where weight management is concerned. Choosing alkaline diets is the only way to live a healthy life, as well as shed those extra pounds.

Alkaline diets require one to follow a lifestyle completely opposite of the high protein low carb diets. The high protein diets leave the person following it fatigued and tired. It is for those who lead a stagnant life and want to shed some weight. But the weight that is lost comes back on as soon as one stops the diet.

With alkaline diets this is not the case. The diets can be incorporated into one's way of life and within days the results start to show. They require one to eat about 80% alkalizing foods so as to maintain the alkaline ph of the body at 7.4.

High protein diets tend to make the ph

of the body acidic as opposed to its natural alkaline tilt. When the body's ph becomes acidic it attracts all kinds of illnesses and depletes one of energy. An acidic ph also results in rapid degeneration of the human body cells. That leads to a shortened life. One should stay away from these crash diets and look at achieving health and vigor by following alkaline diets instead.

Alkaline diets lead to the body's ph maintaining its alkaline nature. The various body functions are carried out smoothly and the immune system of the body stay strong. Under these circumstances one feels energetic as opposed to feeling fatigued. Also the weight shed like this stays off and most importantly the body does not fall sick.

In other words they help repel diseases as opposed to high protein diets which seem to attract them. These plans are also very good for those suffering from chronic diseases like arthritis, cancer, migraines, sinusitis and also osteoporosis. Following such a regime while taking medication helps fight these diseases off from the root.

Alkaline diets constitute mostly of fruits and vegetables. One should try to consume green vegetables and sweet fruits so that they make up about 70 to 80 percent of their total food intake. Lemons and melons should also be eaten. Almonds, honey, and olive oil are also high on the list of foods to be consumed for following alkaline diets.

Meats and fats should be avoided. All

foods that are acidifying like coffee, alcohol, meats, and even certain vegetables like cooked spinach should not form more than 20% of one's diet. Alkaline water is also a must for everyone wanting to improve their diet. At least 6 to 8 glasses of alkaline water can do wonders for your body cleansing. Processed food is all acidic and also high in weight gaining substances and so should be avoided. Beverages like sodas are highly acidic and should not be consumed at all. It takes 32 glasses of water to balance out one glass of soda.

CHAPTER TWO

BENEFITS OF ALKALINE DIETS

Wondering about the benefits of alkaline diets? Then you're not alone, because many people would love to learn more about this healthy way of eating, but they just aren't certain where to begin learning the real deal. That's why I'm giving you a guide to help you learn the truth about what alkaline diets are and the advantages that you can enjoy.

This nutrition program is called several

different names, including the acid alkaline diet, the alkaline diet, and the alkaline ash diet. These names all refer to the same basic concepts, which stress fresh vegetables, fruits, whole grains, legumes, and healthy oils.

Why the Interest in Alkaline Diets?

Scientists realize that the breakdown of foods results in byproducts that can be either acid or alkaline, and that these byproducts can influence acid-alkaline balance in the body. The ideal pH of a healthy body is slightly alkaline, but the more acid-producing foods that are introduced, the more acidic the body becomes. An acidic internal system puts a person at risk for numerous health problems.

A great majority of the foods that the

typical person eats today are highly processed, and they contain high levels of refined carbohydrates, unhealthy fats, sodium, and chemicals that contribute to health concerns. Sweet rolls, meats, and cream cheese all produce many acids when they are digested and absorbed. Processed foods are another type of product that increases the presence of acidic compounds. All of these acids are quickly released into the body's bloodstream, which creates problems as the body struggles to keep up its normally alkaline pH balance.

Experts say that you should have a pH level in the range of 7.35 to 7.45, but with the highly acidic American diet, it is difficult to maintain a healthy pH level, according to alkaline diet experts. These proponents believe that by supporting the body with the type of diet for which it was designed, better health and longer life can be attained. Humans are built for a diet of fresh produce and other whole foods that have been subjected to minimal processing.

What are the Benefits of Alkaline Diets?

According to nutrition experts, it is an acidic diet that is at least partially responsible for common problems such as premature aging and chronic illness. Health conditions such as arthritis and kidney stones are believed to be linked to diets that are known to generate excessive amounts of acids in the body.

Switching to a low-acid diet is believed to be capable of increasing energy, reducing mucus, relieving symptoms of irritability and anxiety, and may even lead to fewer headaches and infections. Scientists are now looking into claims that an alkaline diet has the power to prevent bone loss, muscle wasting, urinary tract problems, and kidney stones.

Ask people who follow these diets, and they'll tell you that they're healthier, happier, and more energetic than their counterparts who follow more low-carb diets. Plenty of people have found that their own health issues have either decreased dramatically or been completely eliminated once they adopted alkaline diets. Losing weight is also an important perk for those who incorporate whole foods into their lifestyles.

How to Get the Most Out of an Alkaline Diet

It can be helpful to refer to a list of specific foods, but generally you should attempt to eat an abundance of fresh fruits and vegetables every day. Salads are always a good choice. Make sure to drink lots of water, vegetable juice, or herbal teas. Avoid processed foods, fried foods, chocolates, foods that contain added sugars, and junk foods. Instead of adding sugar or salt to the foods you cook, try using healthy and flavorful herbs and spices.

The food that we eat today is totally different from what our ancestors ate and is completely different from what we are so accustomed to these days. How aptly said, "We are what we eat." With the advancement of technology, the types of foods we consume make us drag along. A view at the grocery store will shock you with aisles and aisles of processed food items and animal products. With the easy availability of fast foods nowadays, there is no difficulty in finding it in our neighborhoods.

Fad diets are being partly to blame for introducing whole new eating habits, and this includes high-protein diets. In recent years, consumption of animal products and refined food items have increased as more and more people leave out the daily supply of fruits and vegetables in their diets.

It comes as no surprise why, these days, many people are suffering from different types of ailments and allergies such as bone diseases, heart problems and many others. Some health experts link these diseases to the type of foods we eat. There are certain types of food that disrupt the balance in our body so that, during such instances, health problems arise. Unless we modify our eating habits, it's unlikely that prevention of diseases and restoration of health can be achieved.

Why Alkaline Is Important For Our Body

For a healthy body, the alkaline and acid ratio must be balanced, which is measured by the pH level in the body. pH values range from 0 to 14 and 7 is considered neutral. Any value less than 7 is considered acidic. Refined foods, such as meat and meat derivatives, candies and some sweetened drinks usually generate great amount of acid for the body.

Acidosis, a case of high level of acidic in the blood stream and body cells is the common index for the current different diseases inflicting many people. Some health professionals conclude that acidosis is responsible for the critical diseases suffered by many individuals nowadays.

An Alkaline or alkaline diet, which is normally present in our body neutralizes the high level of acid in the body to achieve an equilibrium state. This is the main function of the alkaline in the body. However, the presence of the alkaline in the body is quickly depleted due to the high level of acidic contents it has to neutralize and there is insufficient alkaline food consumed to replenish the loss of alkaline.

A Balanced Alkaline-Acid Level For A Healthy Body

As described previously, acidosis causes many health-related problems. A critical level of acid gets into our system, breaking up the cells and organs when not neutralized properly. To prevent this, one must see to it that a balanced pH is maintained.

To test whether our body contains a higher level of alkaline can be carried out with ease. This is done with the use of pH strips, which are obtainable from any pharmacy. There are two types of strips, one for the saliva and the other for urine.

Generally, a saliva pH level strip will determine the level of acid your body is producing; the normal values should be between 6.5 and 7.5 throughout the day. A urine pH level strip will show the level of acid; a normal reading should be between 6.0 and 6.5 in the morning and between 6.5 and 7.0 at night

High Level of Acidity Is Harmful for the Body

If you consistently suffer from fatigue, headaches and having regular common cold and flu, these symptoms indicate a high level of acid in the body. The effect of acidosis in the body not only inhibits the normal diseases that we know of, but other diseases that you may suffer from are caused by a high level of acid in the body.

Depression, high acidity, ulcers, dry skin, acne and being overweight are some of the things linked with an extreme level of acidity in our body. Not limited to these, there are other critical and serious diseases such as joint diseases, osteoporosis, bronchitis, frequent infections and heart diseases.

Even with medications, the symptoms may be disguised and continue to affect your health as the root of the problem has not been completely eradicated. Taking more medicine will only compound the problem as the anti-inflammatory medicine will add to the acidic level in the body.

Alkaline Diet - A Sure Bet To A Healthy Body

In order to reach the root of the diseases, our system's pH value must be maintained in a healthy state. Naturally occurring alkaline foods are able to supplement the lost alkaline levels in the body during the neutralizing process. By maintaining a healthy alkaline diet, sufficient amounts of alkaline are replenished in the system, thereby bringing the body back to the predominant alkaline state.

So, what are the ways to include an alkaline diet into our eating habits? The very basic first step is to reduce the amount of refined food intake. As we already know, these foods contain many chemicals which are the culprits in increasing the acidic level in our body.

The next step is to cut down on the intake of meat and their derivatives and also the amount of liquor. The final step is to increase the amount of fresh fruits and vegetables, as they are naturally high in alkalinity.

Oranges and lemons are known for being able to convert acidic into alkaline after digestion and are absorbed by the body as part of a good alkaline diet. Generally, we must consume 75% of alkaline food daily. The higher the amount of alkaline foods we put into our system, the greater the neutralization of the acidic condition in our body.

Why It Is Recommended?

If you have heard of the Atkins diet, then the Acid Alkaline Diet is the complete opposite of that. The Atkins diet is a high protein, high fat but low carbohydrates diet. But such diets have a tendency to leave one low on energy and also they seem to be improper gastronomically speaking.

An acid alkaline diet on the other hand is not only useful for weight loss, but over and above that is extremely beneficial to the body's functions. An Acid alkaline, also known as an alkaline ash diet, alkaline acid diet and the alkaline diet, keeps the ph level of the body balanced and so safeguards against various illnesses. Even chronic diseases like arthritis can be not only prevented, but also cured if such a diet is followed.

The basis of a diet that is acid alkaline lies in the fact that our body's ph ideally should be at 7.3. This slightly alkaline level of the body's ph keeps all the vital organs functioning well, as well as the absorption of various minerals is optimized. When this ph tilts to the acidic side trouble starts brewing. An acidic ph level leads to almost all body parts suffering in one way or the other.

Now since our body needs to be alkaline in nature it should reflect in our food intake too. Foods that are alkalizing should be consumed much more as opposed to the acidifying foods. Translated into a simpler language this would mean more vegetable and fruit consumption and very low meats and oil intake.

If the body's alkaline minerals such as calcium, magnesium and potassium levels drop, so will its health, causing it to degenerate and its defenses to drop their guard. An alkaline diet protects that from happening. An acid alkaline or an alkaline ash diet comprises of 80% alkalizing foods and 20 % acidic foods. Since the acid alkaline ratio in the body should be one is to four, our food intake should be of a similar nature.

An alkaline diet is not only recommended to shed those extra pounds, but is also and more importantly a great means of regaining lost health and leading a longer and more disease free life. This diet is especially recommended to those who feel tired most of the time. Stress and a low energy level can both be done away with a diet that is acid alkaline.

Those who suffer from frequent viral

fevers or those who have a nasal congestion most of the time can lead healthier lives if they have a diet that is acid alkaline. Weak nails, dryness, headaches, muscle pain, hives, joint pains, and many more such diseases find their answer in an alkaline ash diet.

A higher level of vegetable intake is recommended in an alkaline ash diet. Lemons should be squeezed into water drinks. Millet or quinoa is preferred over wheat, olive oil over vegetable oil and soups like miso are very useful for following an alkaline ash diet.

Lost health and vigor can be regained and many chronic illnesses prevented as well as cured if an acid alkaline diet is followed. It is a fairly easy diet plan, which should adapt you for a longer and healthier life span.

Benefits of Alkaline Diet for Diabetics

The human body is, to some degree, alkaline by design. By maintaining it alkaline we allow it to run at an ideal level. Nevertheless, millions of reactions of our metabolism yield acidic wastes as end products. When we consume an excessive amount of acid-producing foods and not enough alkaline-forming foods we aggravate the body's acid intoxication. If we let these acid-wastes build-up throughout the body, a disorder known as acidosis develops over time.

Acidosis will progressively debilitate our body vital functions, if we do not quickly take corrective actions. Acidosis, or body over-acidity, is in fact one of the leading causes of human aging. It makes our body highly vulnerable to the series of the deadly degenerative chronic diseases, such as diabetes, cancer, arthritis, as well as heart diseases.

For this reason, the biggest challenge we humans have to face to protect our lives is actually to find the right way to reduce the production, and to maximize the elimination of the body acidic wastes. To avoid acidosis and the age-related diseases, and to continue running at its highest level possible, our body needs a healthy lifestyle.

This lifestyle should include regular exercise, a balanced nutrition, a clean physical environment, and a way of living that brings the lowest stress possible. A healthy lifestyle allows our body to keep its acid waste content at the lowest level possible.

The alkaline diet, also known as the pH miracle diet, seems to fit the best for the design of the human body. This is mainly because it helps neutralize the acid wastes and allows flushing them out from the body. People should look at an alkaline diet as general dietary boundaries for humans to abide by. The persons who have particular health issues and special medical diets might better accommodate those diets to alkaline diet boundaries.

Alkaline Diet Benefits for Diabetics

The miracle alkaline diet will help improve the overall health of the persons suffering from diabetes. As it does for other human beings, an alkaline diet will help boost their body's physiology and metabolism, as well as their immune system. This diet will allow diabetics to have a better control on their blood sugar. It is also going to help not only in reducing their weight gain and the risks of cardiovascular diseases, but also in keeping their cholesterol level low.

In fact, the alkaline diet allows a better management of diabetes and, as a result, it helps diabetics more easily to avoid the degenerative diseases connected to their condition. So by following an alkaline diet, despite their health situation, diabetics can, at the same time, live healthier and extend their life expectancy considerably.

The alkaline diet rule sets general nutritional guidelines. According to this diet plan, our daily food intake should be composed of a minimum of 80 percent of alkaline-forming foods, and of no more than 20 percent of acidifying food products. Additionally, the diet highlights that the more alkaline a food item is, the better it is actually; and on the other hand the more acidifying a food product is, the worse it should be for the human body.

As for the glycemic index rule, it divides foods into four main categories with respect to their ability to raise the blood sugar. This ability is now measured by the glycemic index GI that ranges from 0 to 100. (1) Foods that contain almost no carbohydrates and that have, in consequence, a negligible glycemic index (GI~0); diabetics may take them freely. (2) Foods containing carbohydrates with a low glycemic index (GI 55 or less); people with diabetes should eat these products with some precautions. (3) Foods that have carbohydrates of high glycemic index (GI 56 or more); diabetics must, so far as possible, exclude them from their diet. (4) Processed foods; diabetics will need to consult the manufacturers' labels to figure out their particular glycemic index values.

Diabetics Top Best and Top Worst Foods

Intended for the people affected by diabetes, the 'Diabetics Acid-Alkaline Food Chart' divides foods into six categories. The list below goes from the top best to the top worst foods.

1. Alkalizing food items with GI~0. They are among the top best foods. Diabetics

may eat them freely.

Asparagus; broccoli; parsley; celery; lettuce; carob; vegetable juices; mushrooms; squash; okra; zucchini; cauliflower; garlic/onions; green beans; beets; cabbage; raw spinach; lemons; avocados; limes; goat cheese; herb teas; stevia; lemon water; ginger tea; green tea; canola oil; olive oil; flax-seed oil.

2. Alkalizing food products that have a GI of 55 or less. People who have diabetes should take them with moderation, because of their glycemic index.

Barley grass; sweet potato; carrots; fresh corn; olives; peas/soybeans; tomatoes; bananas; cherries; pears; oranges; peaches; grapefruit; mangoes; kiwi; papayas; berries; apples; almonds; Brazil nuts; wild rice; chestnuts; coconut; quinoa; hazelnuts; lentils; soy milk; soy cheese; goat milk; breast milk; raw honey; whey.

3. Acidifying foods with a GI~0. Diabetics should consume them with caution, being their acid-producing character.

Rhubarb; cooked spinach; pork; shellfish; liver; oysters; beef; venison; lamb; cold water fish; chicken; turkey; eggs; butter; buttermilk; cottage cheese; cheese; corn oil; lard; margarine; sunflower oil; wine; beer; coffee; cocoa; tea; mayonnaise; molasses; mustard; vinegar; artificial sweeteners.

4. Acidifying foods having a GI of 55 or less. Considering both their acid-forming feature and their glycemic index, people with diabetes will need to eat them with

restraint.

Lima beans; navy beans; kidney beans; pinto beans; blueberries; cranberries; sour cherries; prunes; plums; brown rice; sprouted wheat bread; corn; oats/rye; whole wheat/rye bread; pasta/pastries; wheat; walnuts; peanuts; pistachios; cashews; pecans; sunflower seeds; sesame; yogurt; cream; raw milk; custard; homogenized milk; ice cream; chocolate.

5. Alkaline-forming foods with a GI of 56 or more. Because of their high glycemic index, these products are among the worst foods for diabetics. Therefore, people who suffer from diabetes need to avoid them.

Turnip; beetroot; tofu; potato with skins; figs; grapes/raisins; dates; melons;

pineapple; watermelon; rice syrup; maple syrup; raw sugar; amaranth; millet.

6. Acid-producing foods with a GI of 56 or more. These items are too acidic and have too high-glycemic index carbohydrates. They represent the top worst foods for diabetics. Thus, diabetes sufferers need to cut them completely from their meals.

CHAPTER THREE

ALKALINE DIET AND CANCER

As a result of the epidemic of cancer that has broken out in recent years, there have been great strides made in where cancer originated, how it grows in the body and how effective an alkaline diet and cancer regime has become. The definition of cancer allows the patient to have some control in the prevention and battle of cancer cells. By sticking to a primarily alkaline diet, this reduces, and actually quenches, the production of cancer and other diseases. Because of this, an alkaline diet has been found to prevent disease, while an acidic diet encourages disease and cancer to grow.

When you take the definition of cancer simply, it is 'a malformed cell.' This malformed cell can only reproduce malformed cells, and since the human body reproduces tens of thousands of cells daily, the answer is to stop that reproduction. The best defense then is a good offense, and that is what an alkaline diet does as it feeds the good cells, while choking out the disease.

The foods that are taken into the body typically come from two categories - foods that produce an acidic environment and foods that produce an alkaline environment. If you are taking a large quantity of medicines, this might cause your system to lean more towards the acidic, but it can be counteracted by consuming more alkaline-producing foods.

An alkaline diet is generally made up of alkaline-producing foods, so that the pH level is brought to a level of around 7.4. If you search online there are alkaline/acidic charts of all the foods. If you are just beginning this diet, make a copy of the chart and carry it with you when you shop or go out to eat.

In general, stay away from processed foods, fast foods fried in trans fat, any food made with white sugar or white flour, and all foods with chemicals and steroids. These foods all feed cancer cells. If this is what your diet is made up of, check the alkaline food list and see what to be eating now.

Foods on that are alkaline-producing are vegetables, seeds, most fruits, brown rice and other grains, and fish. These foods can be mixed and matched to your own preference for at least 80% of your total diet, and then you add 20% of the acidic-producing foods, and the acidic foods are not all "bad." Foods on the acidic side are whole grain breads, lean meats, milk and milk products, butter and eggs, and this adds up to make an 100% alkaline diet.

To monitor your pH level once you have gotten started on an alkaline diet and cancer fighting way of eating, check any health food store for pH strips or litmus paper. There will be a color chart included to use and determine what your pH blood level is. For an alkaline system, it should register between 7.2 - 7.8. No two people are alike, so test your pH level about once a day as you get started. Then continue to check once a week. If you need to raise your pH level, eat more alkaline foods and use green supplements. An alkaline diet will prevent disease naturally.

Alkaline is most synonymous to its energy producing properties, hence alkaline batteries. It is this same energy generating properties that have been integrated into a diet principle. The alkalizing diet is also known as several other names, such as: ash diet, acid alkaline diet and the alkaline acid diet, is a method of consuming food that will leave ash residue, therefore prompting a process similar to catabolised foods. Catabolise or catabolism simply put is a manner of breaking down molecules into simple waste, therefore creating energy.

While the diet sounds complex in reality it is not. Alkalizing diets revolve around simple rules such as consuming several fresh fruits of the citrus family, legumes, vegetables, tubers, nuts and low sugar based fruits. Just about all the food consumed and digested once released to the blood is either converted into acids or alkaline. Exceptions to the alkalizing diet are fungi, sugar, caffeine and alcohol as well as avoidance of grains. The reason behind this exception is that these foods once digested will turn into acid.

The goal of this diet is to help maintain the body's natural pH level which is around 7.35-7.45. This practice ensures a stable alkalinity in the blood without stressing the body's acid base regulators.

Not to say that the body cannot maintain a pH level without this diet, while our system will automatically do this for us, it is however, maintained at a somewhat respectable level that can easily go from good to better or good to bad. What makes the alkaline diet essential is that it provides the body a different source of minerals like calcium from the bones instead of it having to dip into these said reserves.

As people age the pH balance fluctuates easily and can cause a decline in renal functions and the alkaline diet helps maintain the balance necessary in order to avoid this health decline in the future. Proponents of an alkalizing diet maintain that high acid producing foods can easily disrupts the natural balance, therefore incurring a loss in essential minerals such as magnesium, potassium, sodium and calcium when the body tries to restore its balance. some practitioners attribute this erratic activity towards the cause of illnesses.

Headaches, nasal congestion, sluggishness or lack of energy, anxiety, irritability, excess mucous production, nervousness, cysts, constant colds or flu are symptoms that alkalizing diet practitioners would attribute to a person with an imbalanced alkaline level. The diet is not widely practiced, yet as most physicians do not believe that the reduction of acid containing food such as meats, salts, refined grains and dairies and the increase of an alkaline diet is entirely beneficial to a person's health.

Furthermore, doctors will also point out that they are also uncertain that acids in an individual's diet are the main cause of chronic illnesses as claimed by alkaline diet followers. It is however proven that alkalizing diets do lessen the chances and help prevent osteoporosis, muscle waiting brought about by aging and the buildup of calcium stones in the kidneys.

Way too many people are facing terrible health problems such as cancer, diabetes, liver disease, high blood pressure, and more. Doctors over medicate patients and they become dependent on these medications. It is too bad more people have not heard about the Alkaline Acid Diet. This diet helps you keep an alkaline body and balance your body's pH. This diet is known to have cancer fighting properties and huge health benefits.

Ever wondered why the heart never gets a cancer? The heart might get affected eventually by cancer of any other part of the body, but we never hear of cancer of the heart. This is because the heart never gets cancer. The Alkaline diet is perhaps the only permanent way to prevent and rid oneself of cancer.

Let us understand what causes cancer and how an alkaline diet can prevent it.

Each cell in our body takes in oxygen, nutrients and glucose while it throws out toxins. These cells are protected by the immune system. But as the body gets acidic the immune system gets overpowered by the toxins and the cell loses its capacity to take in oxygen and thus ferments. This cell gets cancer affected and is lost.

The next question is can cancer be prevented and cured by consuming a diet with less acid and more alkaline? Cancer cells lie dormant in a ph of 7.4 but as the body gets alkalized higher and the ph level reaches 8.4, these malignant cells die off. So the answer to cancer lies in an extremely alkaline diet. With the right consumption leading to a high alkaline body ph the cancer cells cannot live in that environment and die off.

Cancer cells being anaerobic cannot live in oxygen. They can only thrive in very low oxygen conditions. When the ph of the body is maintained by consuming an alkaline diet the immune system of the body stays strong. This leads to the cells getting enough oxygen and discarding their toxin waste. Cancer will neither thrive nor take birth under such circumstances.

How does an alkaline diet prevent cancer? Such a diet leads to a high alkaline body ph. This high alkaline body ph results in alkaline tissues in the body. Alkaline tissues hold 20 times more oxygen than acidic tissues.

Cancer cannot live in an oxygenated atmosphere. If the cells are oxygen rich they will prevent cancer. Therefore, while an acidic tissue will be an ideal ground for cancer to develop as well as spread, an alkaline tissue will destroy a cancer cell.

Having a lot of green vegetables and fruits along with alkaline water can save you from cancer. To give your body the best alkaline/acidic balance requires one to eat foods that are highly alkalizing while avoiding the acidifying foods.

An alkaline diet is very beneficial in fighting many diseases apart from cancer. Alkaline supplements are good ways to include alkaline food in your diet. Over cooking of vegetables leads to their nutrients being destroyed. Alkaline supplements make sure one gets enough alkalizing foods in a day. Also, alkaline water is a good alternative to ordinary water. So if you want your body to be cancer free as well as healthy and energetic adopt an alkaline diet and make it your way of life.

CHAPTER FOUR

ALKALINE DIET AND WEIGHT LOSS

What if you knew about a weight loss program that would help you lose weight and feel younger? Would you try it? The alkaline diet and lifestyle has been around for over 60 years, yet many people aren't familiar with its natural, safe and proven weight loss properties!

The alkaline diet is not a gimmick or a fad. It's a healthy and easy way to enjoy new levels of health. In this post you'll learn about what this dietary plan is, what makes it different, and how it can produce life-changing results for you, your waistline and your health.

Are you enjoying a slim and sexy body today? If so, you're in the minority.

Sadly, over 65 percent of Americans are either overweight or obese. If you're overweight, you probably experience symptoms of ill-health like fatigue, swelling, sore joints, and a host of other signs of poor health.

Worse yet, you probably feel like giving up on ever enjoying the body you want and deserve. Perhaps you've been told that you're just getting older, but that simply isn't the truth. Don't buy into that lie. Other cultures have healthy, lean seniors who enjoy great health into their nineties!

The truth is, your body is a brilliantly designed machine and if you have any symptoms of ill-health this is a sure sign that your body's chemistry is too acidic. Your symptoms are just a cry for help. This is because the body doesn't just break down one day. Instead, your health erodes slowly over time, finally falling into 'dis-ease'.

What's wrong with the way you're eating now?

The Standard American Diet (S.A.D.) focuses on refined carbohydrates, sugars, alcohol, meats and dairy. These foods are all highly acid-forming. Meanwhile, despite pleas from the nutritional experts, we simply don't eat enough of the alkalizing foods such as fresh fruits, veggies, nuts, and legumes.

In short, our S.A.D. lifestyle upsets the natural acid-alkaline balance our bodies need. This condition causes obesity, low-level aches and pains, colds and flu, and eventually disease sets in.

We've lost our way. This is where an alkaline diet can help restore our health.

I'm sure you're familiar with the term pH, which refers to the level of acidity or alkalinity contained in something. Alkalinity is measured on a scale. You can take a simple and inexpensive test at home to see where your alkalinity level falls, as well as to monitor it regularly.

Medical researchers and scientists have

known for at least 70 years this lesser-known fact....your body requires a certain pH level, or delicate balance of your body's acid-alkaline levels - for optimal health and vitality.

You might think..."I don't need to know all this chemistry. Besides, what does the proper pH balance and alkalinity matter to me?" I know these were my questions when I first heard about alkaline eating.

We'll use two examples of how acid and alkalinity plays a role in your body.

1. We all know that our stomach has acid in it. Along with enzymes, this acid is essential for breaking food into basic elements that can be absorbed by the digestive tract. What if we didn't have any acid in our stomachs? We would die

from malnutrition in no time because the body couldn't utilize a whole piece of meat or a whole piece of anything, for that matter! Make sense?

2: Different parts of our body require different levels of acidity or alkalinity. For example, your blood requires a slightly more alkaline level than your stomach acids. What if your blood was too acidic? It would virtually eat through your veins and arteries, causing a massive internal hemorrhage!

While these examples demonstrate that the various parts or systems in the body need different pH levels, we don't need to worry about that.

Our problem is simple and it's this.....we are simply too acidic overall, period. If you're interested in learning more about pH you can find tons of information on the web by simply searching the term.

The most important thing to know is this. When your body is too acidic over a long time, it leads to many diseases like obesity, arthritis, bone density loss, high blood pressure, heart disease and stroke. The list is endless, because the body simply gives up the battle for vitality and goes into survival mode as long as it can.

An alkaline diet is unique.

Many diets focus on the same foods that cause you to be overweight or sick in the first place. They simply ask you to eat less of those things, to eat more times per day, or to combine them differently.

In fairness to these diet's creators, they know that many of us don't want to make the bigger changes for our health. We like a diet that's focused on processed and refined foods, our meat, our sugar, alcohols and such. The diet creators are simply trying to help us make easier changes.

We've gotten used to eating this way, and it's not ALL our fault! Greedy food processing giants have a vested interest in keeping us eating this way. Profits are much higher in this sector of the food industry than in the production of your more basic foods like fruits and veggies.

So, again, YES...this diet is different. If those other diets worked you would you would be feeling lean, healthy and vital you wouldn't need to read this article. You wouldn't need a dietary change.

Here's a partial list of foods that you can

eat freely in an alkaline diet:

- Fresh fruits and freshly made juices

- Fresh veggies and juices

- Cooked veggies

- Some legumes and soy

- Lean proteins and some eggs

- Certain grains

- Healthy fats and nuts

*You may be surprised to learn that some veggies and fruits are better for you than others!

You can consume limited quantities of these foods and beverages:

- Dairy

- Many common grains

- Refined foods and sugars

- Alcohol and caffeine

What's it like to be on the alkaline diet, and what results can you expect?

Like any change in diet or lifestyle, you'll go through an adjustment period. Yet because you're burning the cleanest fuel, which your body craves, so unlike many diet plans, you won't ever need to feel hungry. Plus, you can eat all you like until you're satisfied. You also won't need to count calories. And you'll enjoy plenty of variety, so you'll never get bored with eating.

Think of an alkaline diet as a type of 'juice fast' for the body. Only it's not so extreme. You're eating nutrient-dense, easily digestible foods that your body craves. When you provide all the cells of the body that it so desperately needs, your hunger goes away. And there's no need to worry about boring veggies, since there are tons of delicious recipes found on the web and in books.

With all the diet plans out there, why should you consider an alternative plan like the alkaline diet?

When followed properly, you can expect to melt the fat away more easily than with traditional plans. Many testimonials exist where people report losing over two pounds each week. (And that much weight wouldn't be wise in most diet programs.) Plus your skin will become more supple again, your energy will increase and you'll feel younger.

Plus, the alkaline diet does two important things that traditional diets don't.

1. It provides superior nourishment to your body's cells.

2. It naturally helps to detoxify and cleanse the cells, too.

These two facts are behind the reason why an alkaline diet works so quickly and safely.

There are a lot of crazy diets on the market that promise to help you lose weight. Unfortunately, if you look at the nutritional value of some of these diets, they are often severely lacking. If you need to lose weight, you should do it while eating a diet that is good for your body, so that you will become healthier instead of just thinner. An alkaline diet is a healthy approach to weight loss that will keep you energized, healthy, and motivated to drop the pounds.

Understanding the Alkaline Diet

An alkaline diet is different from other diets, because it focuses primarily on the effect that foods have on the acidity or the alkalinity of the body. When foods are digested and metabolized by the body, they produce what is commonly referred to as an "alkaline ash" or "acid ash." The original pH of the food doesn't factor into this final effect within the body.

In fact, some of the most acidic foods such as citrus fruits actually produce an alkaline effect when eaten. When more alkaline foods are eaten as opposed to acid foods, the pH of the body can be adjusted to an optimum level of approximately 7.3. While this is not extremely alkaline, it is enough to reap many healthful benefits.

Using an Alkaline Diet for Weight Loss

Many people attempt fad diets or those which promise quick results in an attempt to lose weight. These diets might produce results in the short term, but over time this can be a very unhealthy way to lose weight. Additionally, many people gain the weight back as soon as they go off their strict diet.

When an acid diet is used for weight loss and control, it is more of a lifestyle change. The results may not happen overnight, but it's more likely that the weight will not be gained back. An alkaline diet is rich in foods which are naturally low in calories, such as most vegetables and fruits.

Many of the foods that are high in fat and calories are also acidifying, so when these foods are removed from the diet, a natural and healthy weight loss will occur. These foods include red meat, fatty foods, high fat dairy products such as whole milk and cheese, sugar, soda, and alcohol.

Once you stop eating these foods, your body will be much healthier, less acidic, and you'll also lose weight in the process. Because the diet is healthy, you can stick with it long term. In fact, many people who start an alkaline diet solely for the purpose of losing weight find many other benefits. An increased energy level, resistance to illness, and an overall improvement in health and well-being are among the many benefits you can experience on an alkaline diet.

How to Start an Alkaline Diet

Many people find that it is easier to start on an alkaline diet by making small changes. Start by slowly reducing the amount of meat, sugar and fat in your diet, while adding fresh fruits, vegetables, healthy fats such as olive oil, almonds, soy products, and natural sweeteners such as Stevia. You'll find over time, your tastes will change and you'll actually start to prefer this kind of diet.

Recently, there have been numerous people claiming that you can use an alkaline diet for weight loss. Is this really true? Can a person really begin to experience weight loss simply from changing their diet to consume more alkaline foods? In this article we're going to show you if alkaline diets are effective, what changes they have on your body, and how exactly to utilize an alkaline diet for your best health.

How Your Body Handles Acid

So, why would anybody care about being on an alkaline diet to begin with? Well the reason is simple. As a population, we are throwing our bodies out of balance by ingesting toxins such as soda and animal proteins in mass quantities. As a result, acid is built up in such large quantities that the body goes into survival mode.

While acid would normally be processed and removed by the liver and kidneys, when too much of it exists, the body stores it in fat in order to preserve the health of your organs. The result is an unbalanced amount of acid and dehydration in the body. The body's homeostasis exists at a pH value of 7.3. Standard (neutral) water has a pH of 7.0. The ability to ionize water and consume an alkaline diet has great benefits for your health.

Alkaline Diet Benefits

But why is an alkaline diet great for weight loss? Well, a myriad of benefits have been attributed to maintaining your body's natural pH. Reversing the effects of chronic diseases such as diabetes, heartburn, angina, migraines, and arthritis are a few of the major benefits.

Freeing diabetics from their insulin crazed hunger fits has resulted in a large amount of weight loss. But, you'll see that even normal people have seen great weight loss as a result of an alkaline diet. When the body is freed of its toxic state, your metabolism is able to function more efficiently. Fat and proteins are burned and stored properly. Also, people have seen the benefits of increased energy and sex drive, allowing them to be more active and productive.

Optimizing Your Alkaline Diet For Weight Loss

If you are attempting to use an alkaline diet for weight loss, it is very important you know how to take the balanced approach. If you use alkaline water and alkaline foods in conjunction with a healthy lifestyle you will receive the "miracle" weight loss that everyone is raving about. Once you begin drinking the alkaline water on a regular basis, you can move from drinking water with pH 9.0 to pH 9.5 (for adults). Consuming a healthy amount of this high pH water is guaranteed to aid the body in returning to acid-alkaline harmony. Also, you should use the high pH water when preparing foods like soup and stews, to balance the acidifying animal proteins or other acidic aspects of the food.

In the above you have seen how you can use an alkaline diet for weight loss, but there is much more to be learned. In order to ensure that you are going to loss weight, it is important you learn about alkaline foods. Some of the most acid filled foods would be the ones you least expect. Many dairy products, for example, are very high in acid content.

Those struggling with excess weight see countless advertisements about thousands of weight loss products. Yet most of these people don't ever know WHY they are overweight in the first place. Many people like to have more energy throughout the day, but the snacks and caffeinated drinks that many consume are highly acid-forming.

What Excess Acidity Does Inside The Body

By creating acidity in blood, tissue and body cells, these typical snacks (as well as fast food, processed food, sweets, all yeast containing products, etc.!) may interfere with healthy energy production and often result in subsequent weight gain. The reason for that is the body's response to excess acidity: it stores acid wastes in fat cells to prevent them from attacking vital organs.

The over-acidification / acidosis of our body cells is the reason for many diseases, will interrupt cellular activities and functions, and is what causes someone to be overweight: to protect itself from potentially serious damage, the body creates new fat cells to store the extra acid. However, as soon as the acidic environment is eliminated, the fat inside the body is no longer needed, and literally melts away.

How To Lose Weight With Alkaline Food?

The body's internal environment is slightly alkaline, which is why it demands a diet that is also slightly alkaline. The body's entire metabolic process depends on an alkaline environment. Our internal system lives and dies at the cellular level, all the billions of cells that make up the human body are slightly alkaline, and must maintain alkalinity in order to function and remain healthy and alive.

Alkaline Food will make food cravings subside naturally, because the acidity inside the internal environment is neutralized through the alkaline forming elements. Once the inner terrain is alkalized with alkaline water and alkaline food according to an alkaline diet (=weight loss diet), the body is free to release the acid waste and burns off fat. In this way, your pH level will also be balanced, and every organ functions better, supporting healthy metabolism and making weight control much easier.

Some Good Alkaline Foods

Fresh vegetables, greens and grasses are excellent anti-yeast and anti-fungal foods, and green grasses such as barley or wheat grass are some of the lowest-calorie, lowest-sugar and most nutrient-rich foods on Earth (and contain high amounts of fiber).

Alkaline foods are mostly vegetables, especially raw ones. Most alkalizing are wheat and alfalfa grasses, fresh cucumber and some kind of sprouts. Furthermore, limes, tomatoes and avocado also have an alkalizing effect to our body, same as most kind of seeds, tofu, fresh soybeans, almonds, or olive oil.

What Are The Results Of The Alkaline

Diet?

Once an alkaline diet is started, most people discover that their pH naturally becomes more alkaline. One gets to see how certain types of meals create a very acidic environment and learn to adjust their eating habits to better support weight control. When pH balance is achieved through alkaline food and alkaline eating habits, the body naturally drops to its healthy weight, food cravings will diminish, blood-sugar levels are balanced and energy levels will increase immensely.

CHAPTER FIVE

ALKALINE WATER

What Is Alkaline Water?

The concept of acidity or alkalinity of the body or of water is based on the pH scale. The pH scale goes from 0 to 14 and a pH of 7 is neutral. Anything with a pH below 7 is considered acidic and anything with a pH above 7 is alkaline.

The acronym "pH" is short for "potential of hydrogen." pH is a measure of the concentration of hydrogen ions. The lower the pH, the more free hydrogen ions it has. The higher the pH, the fewer free hydrogen ions it has. One pH unit reflects a tenfold change in ion concentration, so there are 10 times as many hydrogen ions available at a pH of 7 than at a pH of 8.

Our blood is slightly alkaline, with a pH of 7.4. Pure water has a neutral pH of 7, while natural water ranges from around 6.5 to 8.5 depending on surrounding soil and vegetation, seasonal variations, and weather.

Bottled waters marketed as being alkaline typically claim to have a pH between 8 and 10. Some are from springs or artesian wells that naturally alkaline because of dissolved alkalizing compounds such as calcium, magnesium, potassium, silica, and bicarbonate. Others are transformed by a process called electrolysis that separates the water into alkaline and acid fractions. There are also expensive water ionizing machines marketed for home use.

Why Alkaline Water Cannot Turn The Body Alkaline

Marketers claim that their special water can turn the body alkaline. The truth is that they do not even understand the basic chemistry of how the human body works!

The main reason why drinking alkaline water cannot produce the health benefits claimed by the marketers is because one simply cannot alter the pH of the blood or the body this way.

Our diet, including the water we drink and the medications and supplements we take, can only alter the pH of our urine. Home test kits to measure the pH of urine do not relay any information about the body's pH at all.

The lungs and kidneys are the organs that regulate the body's pH, which is always kept in a very narrow range because all our enzymes are designed to work at pH 7.4. Even a small fluctuation, as little as 0.05 in our blood, can become life-threatening. That is why patients with kidney disease and lung dysfunction often rely on dialysis machines and mechanical ventilators respectively to avoid even a small disruption of pH balance in the blood.

In the stomach, where stomach acid is

secreted, the pH is 1.5 to 3.5. It is a very acidic environment because the acid is necessary to break down the food and to kill all the germs and bacteria that may be in our food.

When we drink alkaline water and it comes in contact with the very acidic stomach, it is immediately neutralized because alkaline water has no buffers. A buffer is a chemical that can react with small amounts of either acid or alkaline substance to prevent changes in pH. An example of an alkaline buffer is baking soda (or sodium bicarbonate). Our lungs use bicarbonate as a pH-stabilizing buffer to maintain a constant blood pH.

Marketers claim that as the stomach acid neutralizes the alkaline water, bicarbonate ions are released into the blood, resulting in an alkalizing effect. This could only be true if the alkaline water effectively neutralized all the stomach acid, like baking soda would have done. But in reality, it is impossible for alkaline water to neutralize any significant quantity of stomach acid to create this "net alkalizing effect". As it happens, it is the other way around, the stomach acid completely neutralizes the alkaline water!

Alkaline Foods And Cancer

Proponents of an alkaline diet and marketers of alkaline water believe that overly acidic diets cause the body to become too acidic, which increases your risk of cancer. Although it is true that the immediate environment around cancer cells can be acidic, do know that it is due to differences in the way tumors create energy and use oxygen as compared to healthy tissues, not the acidic foods (such as meats, dairy, and eggs) that you eat.

Similarly, understand that their proposed answer to increase your intake of healthier alkaline foods like vegetables, fruits, and alkaline water can do nothing to change your body's pH. Veggies are good for you, but for a different reason - they are high in vitamins, minerals, and antioxidants which are anti-inflammatory and cancer-protective.

Alkaline Water For Detoxification And Hydration

Initial health improvements reported by people who drink this type of water can be attributed to the simple fact that they are drinking more water, resulting in improved hydration and detoxification. There is the placebo effect as well.

Moreover, alkaline water may contain higher mineral concentration, which is known to have beneficial health effects, especially when one's diet consists of mainly processed or junk foods that are very low in nutrients.

Alkaline PH-Level

The term pH stands for "potential" of "Hydrogen." It is the amount of hydrogen ions in a particular solution. The more ions, the more acidic the solution. The fewer ions the more alkaline (base) the solution. pH is measured on a scale of 0 to 14 with seven (7) being neutral. The lower the pH number the more acidic it is and the higher the number the more alkaline. For example, a pH-level of 3 is more acidic than a pH-level of 5 and a pH-level of 9 is more alkaline than a pH-level of 6. Drinking alkaline ionized water daily will help to balance and increase the ph-value.

As humans, a normal pH-level of all tissues and fluids of the body (except the stomach) is slightly alkaline. The most critical pH is in the blood. All other organs and fluids will fluctuate in their range in order to keep the blood at a strict pH between 7.35 and 7.45 (slightly alkaline). This process is called homeostasis. The body makes constant adjustments in tissue and fluid pH to maintain this very narrow pH range in the blood.

Diet is probably the most important change. Avoid the over consumption of meat, alcohol, soft drinks, caffeine, coffee, most nuts, eggs, vinegar, sauerkraut, ascorbic acid, cheese, white sugar and medical drugs. Add more ripe fruits, vegetables, bean sprouts, water, milk, onions, figs, carrots, beets, and miso to your diet.

Testing the pH Level

Testing saliva is the most effective way to gauge the body's pH. To test saliva: Wait 2 hours after eating. Spit into a spoon. Dip the strip. Read immediately. Use the color chart from the correct indication. An optimal reading is 7.5. This indicates a slightly alkaline body.

To test urine: Test a urine sample first thing in the morning. Fill a small cup with urine, and dip a strip into the cup. Read immediately. Results: 7.0 is neutral. A reading of 6.5 is slightly acidic. A reading below 6.5 is very acidic. Note: A reading of 8.0 or above, while common, indicates a body that is too alkaline. Urine is slightly more acidic than saliva. [from pH strip producer: Phion, Inc.]

About Balancing the pH

People with painful deposits anywhere in their feet may have a morning urine pH of 4.5! At 4.5 it may be safe to guess that a lot has precipitated again in the night. During the day, your body's pH may swing back and forth. The urine gets quite alkaline right after a meal; this is called the alkaline tide. Three meals a day would bring you three alkaline tides. During these periods, lasting about an hour, you have an opportunity to dissolve some of your foot deposits. But if you allow your pH to drop too low in the night you put the deposits back again. The net effect decides whether your deposits grow or shrink.

Items traditionally used to help nutritionally support the normal pH level of the body. The use of these items is a traditional use that is not intended to be prescribed for, to treat or claim to cure any disease, including diseases related to high or low pH levels. To alkalinize yourself at bedtime, choose one of these options:

Take calcium (pure calcium carbonate or coral calcium) equaling 750 mg plus 300 mg of magnesium oxide. The magnesium helps the calcium dissolve and stay in a solution. Taking more calcium at one time is not advised because it cannot be dissolved and absorbed anyway and might constipate you. For the elderly only one calcium tablet is advised. Take calcium tablets with vitamin C or lemon water to help dissolve (1/4 tsp. vitamin C powder; adding honey is fine).

One cup of sterilized milk or buttermilk, drunk hot or cold, plus 1 magnesium oxide tablet, 300 mg. (adding cinnamon is fine). If these two remedies work for you, your morning urinary pH will come up to 6.0, but if for some reason they don't, you may need to take more drastic measures. Take the supplements and milk earlier in the day and reserve bedtime for:

Get Balanced Bicarb Antacid (made from two parts baking soda and one part potassium bicarbonate). This potion may also be useful in occasional allergic reactions. Take 1 level tsp. in water at bedtime. If your pH reaches 6 in the morning continue each night at this dose. If it does not, take 1 1/2 tsp. Keep watching your pH, since it will gradually normalize and you will require less and less.

This is a short list of alkaline foods for pH balance:

Lemons/ Watermelon - pH 9.0

Bell pepper, kelps, mango, melons, parsley, papaya, seaweeds - pH 8.5

Apples, apricots, grapes, fruit juice, avocados, bananas, vegetable juice, peas - pH 8.0

Mushrooms, onions, almond, egg yolks, tofu, soy milk, vinegar, tomato, cucumber, coconut, brown rice - pH 7.5

These are a few common things that leave an acid ash in the bloodstream:

- Most tap water - pH 7.0

- Distilled water - pH 6.5

- Purified water, fruit juice with sugar, cigarette, tobacco, wine - pH 6.0

- White rice, beef, white flour, sugar, yogurt (sweetened) - pH 5.5

Acid pH:

- Reverse Osmosis Water, coffee, white bread - pH 4.0

- Cola, soft drinks, beer, hard spirits - pH 3.0

- Car battery acid - pH 1.0

Acid producing activities and emotions:

Overwork, anger, fear, jealousy, stress physical, stress emotional, Alkalize your body with alkaline diets and alkaline water.

- Stick to alkaline diets while minimizing intake of acid-forming foods

- Eat more greens and reds

- Drink at least 1.5l alkaline water every day

- Aerobic activities, yoga, tai chi, walking, swimming, rebounding and a positive mind are alkaline inducing.

Keep the body in an optimal healthy state:

1) The acid-alkaline balance, or pH balance or Yin-Yang balance in terms of

Traditional Chinese Medicine, of the body is critical to optimal health. It is said that Taoists, Qigong masters and Yogis all live a balanced, harmonized and alkaline life. Acidified body, imbalance, and physical weakness caused by poor diet and soft drinks, stress and toxic environment are very common among most Americans.

Microstructure, electron-rich, reducing alkaline water is the smallest antioxidant in molecular size, thus drinking alkaline water is the simplest and most effective way to neutralize free radicals, acidic waste and carcinogen and flux out the accumulated toxins which are all electron-loving and provide best hydration to each cell in the body.

Positive effects of being alkaline and

hydrated:

2) Blood is one of the fluid systems that are constantly trying to maintain a pH of 7.4 (slightly alkaline). Being slightly alkaline means the blood cells and body tissues are highly oxygenated, and in optimal state to neutralize and detoxify the metabolic waste and toxins and you will be in a state of:

- Vibrant healthy body

- Enhanced immunity

- High energy level

- Sharp mind and brain performance

- Shining looking healthy skin

- Positive emotional state

The pH balance is one of the most important measures to avoid disease at first and build up a strong functioning immune system. Cancer patients for example are always toxic (without exemption!) and most of the time eating the wrong food and having emotional stress or other stress related issues.

Terrain refers to the environment, the body fluids, humors. These make up 80% of the body and need to have a pH value of 7,2-7,6 so that the protits take on the form of life-supporting bacteria. Due to interruptions in Meridian Energy flow pH values can be different in various parts of the body. When the pH value changes the protits change into bacteria that can live in this low-pH, acicity environment.

Environment has 2 causes, Metabolism and Energy, both are interchangeable as 1st and 2nd causes. Protits are indestructible, they change their life forms = Pleomorphism. Energy is indestructible = change of flow in meridians.

For example, cholera bacteria requires pH 6 (assumed figure for demonstration purposes).

Cholera bacteria enters the body, which has 7.2 Protit will now change to a form that can live in 7.2, hence no outbreak of cholera. If body is at 6 cholera bacteria will florish, other bacteria in the body now also changes to cholera bacteria. That's the reason why some people get it and some don't. To explain the correlation between Metabolism and Meridian Energy which are responsible for the Terrain is a 100+ hour lecture.....

Nothing is a secret. 'Merck et al tests'

every new antibiotic against its pleomorhic effect, so they know into what kind of bacteria the cholera will change (another harmful one as it lives in the same pH 6 environment). They know the only cure is to change the Terrain to pH 7.2, but this can only be done by metabolism, which requires good food and an undisturbed flow of energy. >>

Pulsating Energy Resoance Therapy (PERTH):

- Energy buildup and meridian (organ) balancing (PERTH)

- Complete body detoxification - naturally and soft

- pH normalization

- Treatment & Prevention of over 200

dis-ease conditions

- Increased cell metabolism

- Blood pressure normalization

CHAPTER SIX

EATING ALKALINE FOODS

To become healthy you have to think healthy and this is why many people these days are turning to alkaline food diets. This is excellent for both your health and for your body. People on this diet have claimed they not only feel good, but also have more energy, an improved digestion and much less mood swings than before they started.

What Is an Alkaline Diet?

An alkaline diet is basically eating alkaline foods. The foundation for this diet is vegetarian. To get the best from this diet we will give you some guidance below.

- Vegetables would be arguably the most alkaline food around. Easy to buy and easy to prepare.

- Try to choose whole grain foods rather than processed ones because processed products do not have the same nutritional content.

- Some acidic foods such as limes, lemons and grapefruits turn to alkaline after digestion, so are very useful for flavouring.

- Other acidic foods also able to be used in this diet are coffee, cola, and broccoli, artichoke, asparagus, beetroot, spinach and cauliflower.

- Avocado, celery, garlic, ginger, onions, pumpkin are ideal vegetables to include.

- Tomatoes, pears, papayas, mango, apricots and apples can be included.

- Nuts to use are sunflower seeds, almonds, and walnuts.

- Oats, brown rice, and also almond and brown rice milks as well as coconut and coconut water can also be used.

Foods to Avoid

Red meat, poultry, dairy products and fizzy drinks are the foods that are the hardest to digest. Your kidneys have to take minerals which are vital for the body, like calcium and magnesium, from the bones in order to dissolve the acid in these foods.

This is not to say that small quantities of the above cannot be used to supplement and add variety to your meals. You will soon realise exactly what you can and cannot use, as your body will soon tell you.

Move towards this alkaline diet gradually. If you eat a lot of meat or love dairy foods like cheese, it may be best to try an alkaline diet meal 3 times a week to start with, so your body does not go into shock. Any diet has to be approached gently and once your body accepts the new foods being offered it will thank you by looking and feeling good.

As a guideline the pH of alkaline in our

blood is measured from 7.35 to 7.45, and the level of acid is from 1.0 to 9.0.

Alkaline Diet Menu

By consciously controlling the acid to alkaline balance in your body, you are able to benefit from a wide range of health benefits. Increased energy and weight loss will be immediately noticeable to someone who is recently returning to balance from an overly acidic body.

By composing your diet of approximately 80% alkaline foods and only 20% acidic foods, you can return your body to its healthy, natural state. Also, preparing the acidic foods with alkaline water can greatly reduce their acidifying effect on the body. An alkaline diet works to reduce the stress placed on your liver, kidneys, and other organs by having an overly acidic (toxic) body.

Your Alkaline Diet Menu

Below are lists of different foods which are our top recommendations for having an alkaline diet. While foods which are acidic must be ingested for a healthy diet, they are too be lowered back to the levels which our bodies originally adapted to.

Alkaline Fruits:

- apples

- bananas

- blackberries

- dates

- oranges

- pineapple

- raisins

Alkaline Vegetables:

- broccoli

- cabbage

- carrots

- cauliflower

- celery

- eggplant

- mushrooms

- squash

- turnips

Acidic foods should make up no more than 25% of your diet. Listed below are the types of food which are acidic. Keep in mind that every category listed below has foods which are horribly acidic, but also some which are much more on the alkaline side.

Acidic Foods:

- meat

- cheese

- legumes

- grains

- nuts

- select fruits

- select vegetables

Top 10 Healthiest Alkaline Diet Foods

Ever heard of alkaline diet foods? If not, it is high time you do. Work pressure, home making, as well as maintaining personal and professional relations is taking a toll on everyone's food habits, resulting in more than 70% of the present generation suffering from acidity and heartburn. Every third person seems to be complaining of gastric problems, indigestion and acid reflux.

All of this is due to the imbalance in the acid-alkaline pH of foods that are consumed these days, where you simply grab something and rush to work. Fast foods, sodas and the like are being consumed left, right and center by the young generation, thus giving rise to deficiency in minerals, vitamins and nutrition.

Alkaline diets have been found to be extremely beneficial for optimum health. You can keep chronic ailments such as acidity, osteoporosis, and generalized weakness at arm's length with foods rich in alkaline content. Alkaline foods are important since the pH of human blood is slightly more alkaline. This makes it necessary that we have more of alkaline pH than acidic content in the body.

What are the benefits of Alkaline Diets?

Alkaline diet foods have a plethora of benefits such as:

- Improved resistance
- Vibrant temperament
- Increased Alertness
- Strong teeth and Bones
- Easy Digestion

Alkaline diet foods are vital to maintain the pH levels of blood at an optimum of 7. Alkaline foods are mostly vegetarian foods consisting of fresh foods and vegetables.

Listed here are the top 10 healthiest alkaline foods for nutritional benefits:

- Spinach and Greens - Spinach has been found to contain maximum benefits and is highly alkaline. It can be consumed raw or cooked with equal effect. Other leafy green vegetables such as lettuce, fenugreek leaves, basil, etc. also are extremely good as alkaline foods. They also contain a lot of minerals and vitamins as an added advantage.

- Cucumber - Raw cucumber is not only a zero-calorie vegetable, it is highly alkaline when consumed raw. It is delicious and contains a host of nutritional benefits. Cucumber improves overall digestion and keeps your skin fresh and glowing. It contains healthy alkaline water that helps in flushing out unwanted wastes from the body.

- Banana - Bananas can be considered a whole food due to its numerous dietary advantages. It gives instant energy and is hugely alkaline. In fact, if you are suffering from severe acidic problems, a banana diet can work wonders in reducing the burning sensation and indigestion remarkably. Bananas have healthy sugar content and can be consumed by anyone irrespective of his health condition.

- Celery - Celery is a delicious alkaline food that can help you immensely in keeping your pH levels at normal range of 7. When half-cooked, it gives maximum nutritional value and can be eaten as fresh salad too.

- Broccoli - Broccoli is one of the most nutritious and alkaline foods that has proved itself time and again. It is easily digestible and is a rich source of valuable minerals such as carotene and calcium. These minerals help in improving immunity and combat diseases in a remarkable manner.

- Avocado - This wonder fruit is a rich source of alkaline food and has an overall benefit in maintaining good health. Avocado improves your hemoglobin content and is extremely beneficial in restoring normalcy in a disease affected body.

- Capsicum - Capsicum, also known as bell pepper is a rich antioxidant and can be useful whether eaten cooked or raw. It is not only of high alkaline and nutritional value, it is also very delicious and adds taste to any dishes that are prepared with capsicum for flavor.

- Potato Skin - Although potato is found to be acidic in nature, potato skin is very rich in alkaline content. Raw potato juice is found to be very useful in reducing the acidic content in the stomach.

- Soy beans - Soy beans and soy milk are greatly alkaline and can be used as nutritional alkaline foods.

- Cold Milk - Cold milk is found to have high alkaline content and is often recommended to combat heartburn and acid reflux disorders.

CHAPTER SEVEN

ALKALINE DIET RECIPES

1. ALKALINE 'ACTIVATOR' GREEN SMOOTHIE

Ingredients:

– 1 lime

– 2 apples, chopped

– 1 inch slice of cucumber

– 1/2 celery stick

– Handful of spinach or kale

– 1 inch slice of pineapple,

– wheatgrass powder, 1 teaspoon

– water, as desired to thin consistency

-1/2 tsp spirulina powder, (optional)

-1/2 avocado, (optional)

Method:

Wash ingredients, place all in blender. Blend, pour, drink, enjoy! Activate your body's energy

Serves 1 (350 calories or 450 with avocado)

2. CREAMY DELICIOUS ALMOND MILK

Ingredients:

– 50g almonds or sliced almonds (it's best if you've soaked them for a few hours beforehand)

– 1 litre filtered water

– 1 tsp sunflower lecithin granules (optional)

– 2 medjool dates with stones removed (optional)

– a few drops of vanilla extract (optional)

Method:

Put all the ingredients in your high speed blender and blend for 1-2 minutes. Pour the milk through a straining cloth and into a container.

Store the milk in the fridge – it will keep for up to three days.

You can use the almond pulp left over in the straining cloth to add into cake or brownie mixes.

Makes 1 litre (350 calories total)

3. CHIA CARDAMOM BREAKFAST PUDDING

Ingredients:

– 50g chia seeds

– 4 cardamom pods

– 10g hemp seeds

– 10g almond flakes

– 200ml almond milk

– 1 tbsp. agave syrup

– A few goji berries for decoration

Method:

Put all ingredients (except the gojis) in a bowl and mix thoroughly until all the chia seeds are covered well with the almond milk. Leave for an hour or two overnight so that the chia seeds expand

and go gelatinous.

Remove cardamom pods and top with the goji berries. Serve and enjoy.

Serves 1-2 (400 calories total)

4. ALKALINE MINT-CHOOCLATE ICE CREAM SMOOTHIE

Ingredients:

– 4 very ripe, frozen bananas

– 4 small dates or 2 large medjool dates

– 1 tsp of carob powder

– 200ml almond milk

– A few sprigs of fresh mint leaves

Method:

Put all ingredients in a high speed blender and blend for 1-2 minutes. Add more almond milk for a thinner consistency or less milk for a thicker ice cream.

Garnish with a sprig of mint.

Serves 1-2 (600 calories total)

5. CREAMY KALE SALAD WITH AVOCADO AND TOMATO

Ingredients:

– 2 large handfuls kale

– 1 ripe medium avocado

– 2 ripe tomatoes

– Juice of 1 lime

– 1 clove crushed garlic or 1/2 tsp garlic powder

– 1 tbsp. agave syrup or honey

– 1/2 tsp. of paprika

1/2 tsp. ground black pepper

Method:

Wash and roughly chop the kale and tomatoes. Place in a large glass or mixing bowl.

Peel the avocado and add to the bowl. Juice the lime and add all remaining ingredients to the bowl. Massage all the ingredients together. Serve and enjoy.

Serves 1-2 (400 calories total)

CBD Oil 2019: What Is All the Hype About?

Get Rid of All the Misconceptions about Hemp and Marijuana, learn what to Look for when Buying CBD, and how does it Help with Different Ailments.

Included: Log Book to Find Your Proper Dosage!

By

Caro Mollet

accurate, up to date, and reliable, complete information. No warranties of any kind are declared or implied. Readers acknowledge that the author is not engaging in the rendering of legal, financial, medical or professional advice. The content within this book has been derived from various sources. Please consult a licensed professional before attempting any techniques outlined in this book.

By reading this document, the reader agrees that under no circumstances is the author or publisher responsible for any losses, direct or indirect, which are incurred as a result of the use of information contained within this book, including, but not limited to, errors, omissions, or inaccuracies.

Hemp vs. Marijuana:

Unless it is otherwise noted, we mainly talk about CBD oil from Hemp. Which has more CBD than the one from the Marijuana plant and less than 0.3 % THC in it. Check out the 2018 Farm Bill for the legalization of Hemp on a federal level.